5:2 AND TRAINING
Learn the benefits of the 5:2 Diet with exercise advice designed to make you feel good.

Live Longer, Be Healthier!

(You need the digital version in PDF to read all the info from the links)

Published by Niclas Brunnegård
Copyright © 2014

http://www.mryeah.com, niclas@mryeah.com

Cover and internal design © MrYeah.com

Copyright & Disclaimer

The information provided in this book is designed to provide helpful information on the subjects discussed. This book is not meant to be used, nor should it be used, to diagnose or treat any medical condition. For diagnosis or treatment of any medical problem, consult your own physician. The publisher and author are not responsible for any specific health or allergy needs that may require medical supervision and are not liable for any damages or negative consequences from any treatment, action, application or preparation, to any person reading or following the information in this book. References are provided for informational purposes only and do not constitute endorsement of any websites or other sources. Readers should be aware that the websites listed in this book may change.

Table of Contents

ACKNOWLEDGMENTS 1

DISCOVERING THE 5:2 DIET 2
THE DOCUMENTARY 3
MY BEFORE & AFTER 4
HELPING YOU REACH YOUR GOALS 5
   Recipes...5
   Exercises 5
MY WEBSITE 6

INTRODUCTION 7
WHAT IS THE 5:2 DIET? 7
WHAT DO I NEED TO GET STARTED? 8
HOW DOES 5:2 WORK? 9

BENEFITS 11
LIVE LONGER! LIVE HEALTHIER! (WITH 5:2 DIET) 12
   Future Studies in Progress...13
LIVE LONGER! LIVE HEALTHIER! (WITH 5:2 WORKOUT) 14
AGE 60+: LIVE LONGER AND HEALTHIER, TOO!..15

SIDE EFFECTS 16

WHO SHOULDN'T 5:2 17

5:2 BASICS 18
START EASY 18
TIPS TO SUCCEED 19
HOW QUICKLY WILL I SEE RESULTS?..20
OTHER WAYS TO GET IN SOME EXERCISE- YOU WON'T BELIEVE! 21

MENUS 22
MEAL PLAN #1...22
MEAL PLAN #2...24
MEAL PLAN #3...25
MEAL PLAN #4...26
MEAL PLAN #5...27

WORKOUTS 28
WEEK 1 29
   Pass 1. "10-1"..29
   Pass 2. "3x5"...29
   Pass 3. "550"...29
WEEK 2 30
   Pass 1. "20-15-10"..30
   Pass 2. "20-10"...30
   Pass 3. "10-20-30"..30
WEEK 3 31
   Pass 1. "10-1, 1-10"..31
   Pass 2. "20x5"...31
   Pass 3. "3x5"...31
WEEK 4 32
   Pass 1. "300"...32
   Pass 2. "3x2"...32
   Pass 3. "Go 50!"..32

Acknowledgments

I have much thanks to Dr. Mosley and his documentary. Without his quest to find a healthy and exciting lifestyle change to become healthy and lose weight, I would have never found my happiness!

Many thanks to my lovely, beautiful, and dedicated wife, Sofia, who has given me support and has helped me through this journey. Without her I couldn't have accomplished so much. Thank you.

To my wonderful boys, Alvin and Max, I love you.

Thank you to my trainer, Michael Hansson Sjöö. For you have provided me with so much information. Thank you for working so hard with me.

To my friends.

My editor, Marta Khan, for helping me find my voice in writing. Thank you.

"'There is nothing else you can do to your body that is as powerful as fasting."
-Dr. Michael Mosley medical expert interviewee

Discovering The 5:2 Diet

I got into a viscous cycle of feeling crappy—not healthy at all! If you are like me, then you may have learned how a sedentary job and a lack of desire to exercise can cause you to gain weight. I loved to play football (aka; soccer) but hadn't played in three years. *I missed my health!* So, I decided to play football again. On a Monday in March, I sat benched during a game when I realized that I needed to lose the 8kg (17.6lbs) I had gained during my last viscous cycle. I didn't know where to begin with losing weight; to lose weight and feel healthy, *diet and exercise is everything!*—or is it?

During my research for finding the best methods to get healthy again, I saw a BBC documentary by Dr. Michael Mosley titled, "Eat, Fast, & Live Longer," (http://www.dailymotion.com/embed/video/xvdbtt) in which he tested different methods to **live longer, stay younger, and lose weight** with as little change as possible in his lifestyle. In the documentary, Mosley spearheaded his research and was surprised over his results and test values. Once he tried a diet, what he calls the 5:2, which is a modified version from his research, he was shocked at his results, so he concluded that the 5:2 diet would be sustainable in the long term. The 5:2 diet consists of 5 days of regular eating with 2 days of fasting—or low calorie eating.

After seeing that documentary, I knew immediately that I had to try this 5:2 approach. The research and evidence was compelling in the documentary. I bought Dr. Michael Mosley's book *The Fast Diet* (available with U.S. measurements or in metric measurements) and dove in, pulling ahead and gathering useful recipes. As early as two weeks after, I lost 3kg (6.6lbs) and was amazed. Michael was right! This is life changing!

I want to share with the world, as Michael has to inspire and help you as this helped me. The 5:2 diet is really unique because it isn't only about weight loss but improved health in many, many ways. It also isn't a new way of thinking, or a "fad" diet as many proclaim, but a researched and truly ancient method of human science. I hope this eBook helps guide you in understanding how simple, yet how effective, this ancient and evolved way of feeding the body is. This eBook will help you begin your journey and achieve the body **you deserve!**

To really feel the effects of the 5:2 diet, you owe it to yourself to stick with it for at least 2-3 weeks.

Make that promise to yourself and you'll feel and SEE the difference!

The Documentary

If you have some time, I strongly encourage you to watch "Eat, Fast, & Live Longer". I am providing a link here (http://www.dailymotion.com/embed/video/xvdbtt) and below in the picture, but if this link no longer works, please do an internet search and you will most likely find Dr. Mosley's documentary on DailyMotion, Vimeo, etc. Dr. Mosley is waiting to tell you his **life-changing** discovery! Don't wait to watch it—your health shouldn't have to wait either.

It is _worth_ seeing!

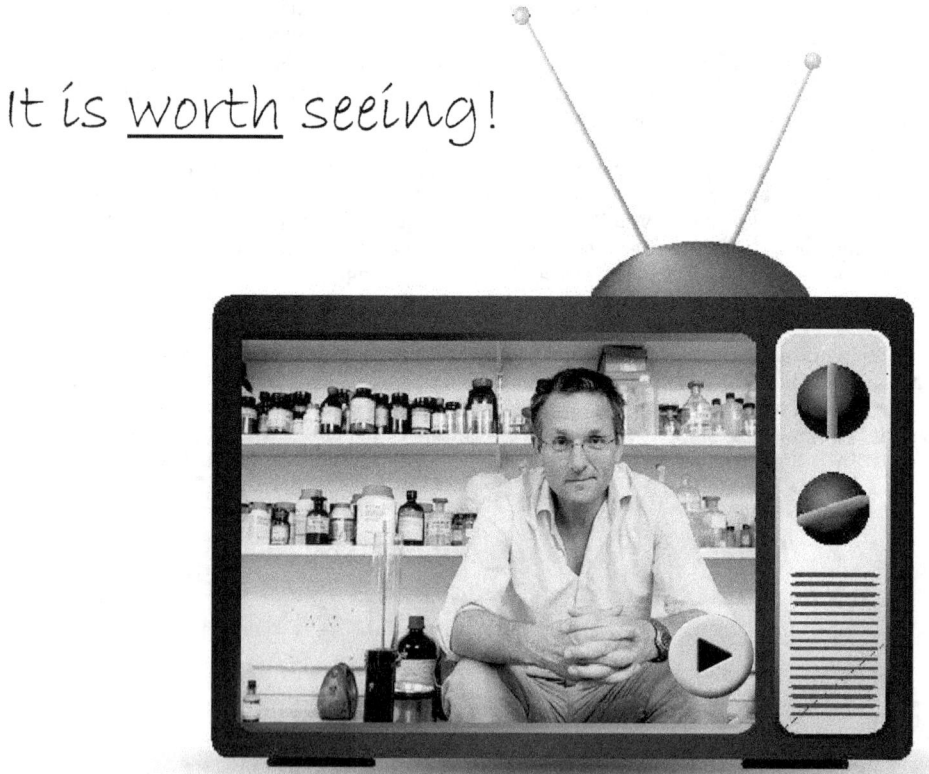

My Before & After

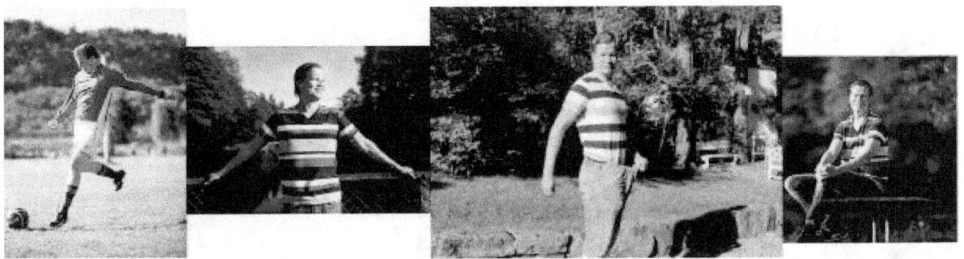

My passion is to help people get started with the 5:2 diet. I believe in the concept and the results. After 7 weeks of being on 5:2, I lost 7kg (15.4lbs). My beer stomach disappeared and I started playing football again—at 38 years old! I felt healthy and alive. The method fits perfectly into my lifestyle. I am married to my wonderful wife, Sofia. We have two boys. I love my lifestyle now and I want you to feel the same way. I want no one to miss this lifestyle! No one. **That means you!** Imagine what better health can do for you? 5:2 revolutionized a family man like me. I feel fantastic now.

I am so excited to help you feel fantastic with this eBook. I also have a website, Mr. Yeah.com, with a forum, a web app, apps that you can download for your smartphone (Apple, Android, search for 5:2-app in the stores), and a Facebook page (https://www.facebook.com/mryeaahhh); these tools will guide you in the beginning and beyond.

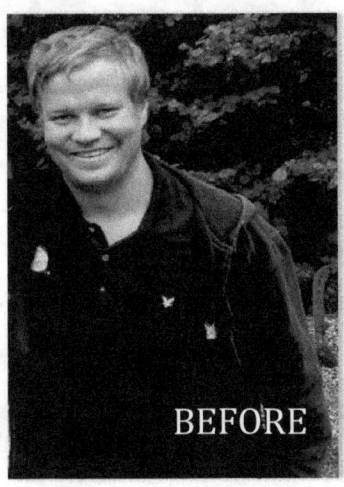

BEFORE

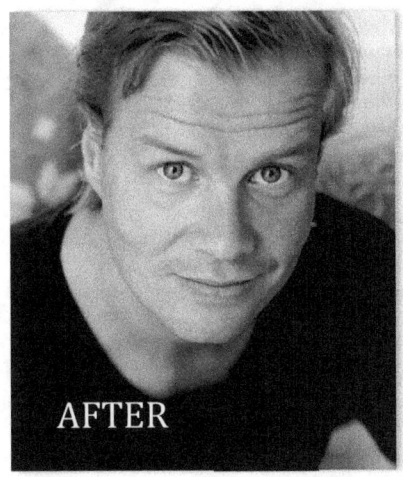

AFTER

4

Helping You Reach Your Goals

Recipes

To help you **reach your goals**, I am providing tried-and-true recipes from my family. I have self-tested recipes together with my wife, Sofia. We test and test, so we know what will make you feel great during the fasting day and provide you a menu that is correctly balanced regarding nutrition and proteins.

The recipes are categorized into menu plans to help you know what to eat throughout a fasting day, but for ultimate success, I recommended that you do a bit of research and find additional recipes that you prefer to add to your cooking collection. The recipes included here are relevant to my culture and country, Sweden, so please, use these recipes as guidelines and feel free to substitute within your own culture's variances—the only thing I ask of you is to watch the nutrition information of your substitutions.

Most foods have nutrition labels, if you are unsure of how these work for you the FDA (Food & Drug Administration) has a great interactive website and quick tutorial called, Make Your Calories Count, that will explain it all for you! **The more you teach yourself, the easier the lifestyle change will occur!**

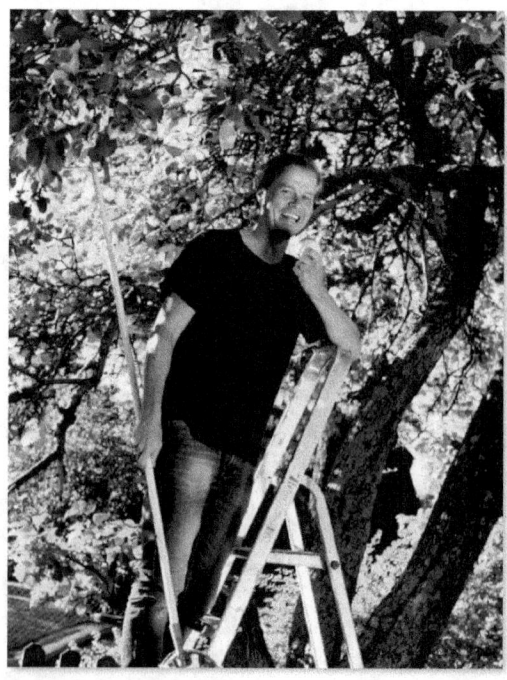

Exercises

To help you reach your goals and **become healthier and stronger**, I have created an exercise program with my personal trainer, Michael Hansson Sjöö. *We call it the 5:2 Workout.* This can be found on the web link, so you can have it on any device as well as in this eBook.

5:2 Workout is a system that consists of three exercise sessions per week. The passes are short and highly intensive and include heart rate-based strength training. The idea is that we will become stronger as our fitness improves.

Three times a week is enough.

5:2 And Training

My Website

I have become so charged by 5:2 that I really want to use my knowledge and experience with it to help people in the world. Sounds extreme? Perhaps, but thanks to this attitude, I have already helped many to start and I get emails every day about how well things are going.

Before 5:2 changed my life, I had the domain mryeah.com for my Premier League football. But, it had never happened. Then 5:2 happened! I decided to post my 5:2 results on the site. I weighed myself every week and measured the waist circumference. Then, I started to write little posts about my experience...I got more and more readers. The media even got in touch! Now, it has become a big thing and I have been in several magazines such as Expressen and Aftonbladet , and newspapers such as, Country and Boras Courier. I decided that I wanted to be even more public with this because **it's an incredible, transforming, yet simple lifestyle**. To Dr. Michael Mosley and 5:2 diet, I owe so very much!

I've mentioned already that I've created a forum for you on my website, Mr.Yeah.com. My site is in Swedish but you can use the droplist to have it translated. If you have difficulties with the droplist, Google has a translation page that will translate any website for you by simply adding text or the webpage address. The forum might be in Swedish but it doesn't matter; you can still ask me in English there. Also, you can email me at niclas@mryeah.com and right quickly get an answer, if you have any questions, or ask me on Facebook.

My goal was not primarily to lose weight, but for all the other health benefits that I will describe. If the goal for you is to lose weight, chances are that you will do so if you follow my advice in this eBook.

I want you to understand how simple this is.

My website,
Mr. Yeah.com

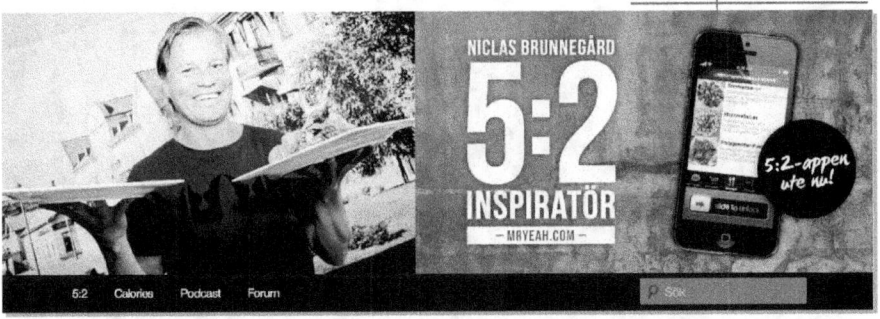

Introduction

What is the 5:2 diet?

5:2 is a diet where you "fast" for 2 days and eat normally for 5 days; this is called "intermittent fasting" or sometimes "calorie restriction". On a fasting day, you do get to eat, but within a restricted calorie amount. Women should get about 500 calories and men about 600. Don't worry! This seems like a small amount but I have a great menu for you to follow that will help you feel well during these fasting days. You don't need to fast for more than 2 days. 2 days is plenty. The next 5 days are all yours!

The best thing about 5:2 is that most people might assume that on those 5 days you would gorge yourself on food, but actually you find yourself eating smaller portions- thus helping in the total outcome! But, losing weight is just one benefit; there are many more benefits that will transform your overall health! Continue reading to learn how 5:2 can increase live span, delay cancer and Alzheimer's, decrease blood sugars, insulin, pressure, and cholesterol! Don't believe it? It's true. People have lived in this mode of eating for thousands of years before the recording of time. Centarians live in all places in the world where diet are restricted[1]—maybe it is time we consider why.

*I believe in the concept of doing 5:2 for 5 months and then changing it to only fasting for 1 day a week, called 6:1. The **5:2 Workout** that we created is well suited to do at home and takes only 15-20 minutes to do...3 times a week. If you follow the 5:2 method, you will lose weight, gain better health values, reduce the risk of cancer, become more alert, sharper, and perhaps even smarter.*

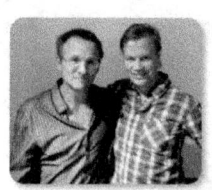

What do I need to get started?

- A kitchen scale
- Proper Food
- 2 days a week

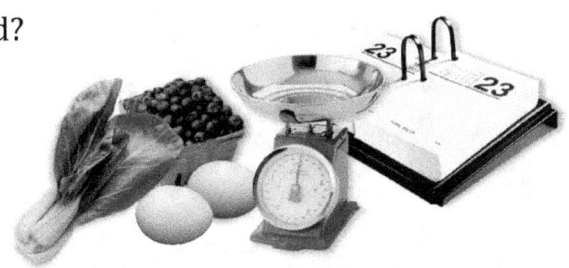

That's it! Then you will buy your foods and weigh them following my recipes. After a while, you will be able to create your own recipes that work best for you. Use my 5:2-app that you can download for your smartphone (Apple, Android to get started). **It couldn't be easier!**

Do you want to replace something or compose your own menu? I have a kcal table (calorie counter) HERE, but you may have to translate my page by using the droplist at http://mryeah.com/ or by using Google Translate.

The strength of this 5:2-app is that we have been testing recipes for a long time so that YOU will really feel good during your fasting day. You will also get nutritious food and proper distribution of proteins.

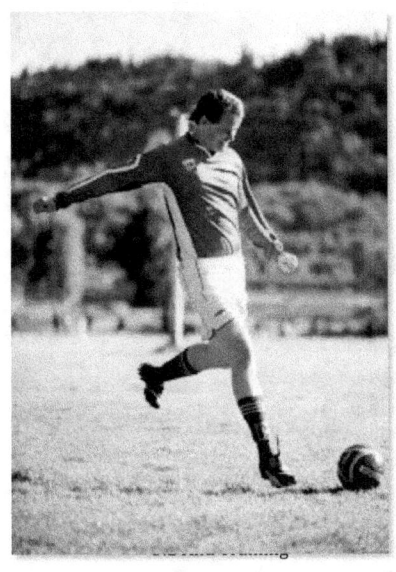

5:2 and high-intensity exercise changes your life! You can do "fat-blasting", "disease reversing" exercises in short amounts of time (even 60+ years old) with HIT (high-intensity training) and super-charge your 5:2 goals! Read more to learn about high-intensity workouts.

That's me after 5:2! Happy again. ☺

How does 5:2 work?

The 5:2 diet is based upon the principal of intermittent fasting, or called calorie restriction. When Dr. Michael Mosley set out on his discovery, his intention was to find a healthy way of lowering weight, blood pressure, cholesterol, and blood sugar, as he was becoming diabetic. He set out across America to learn about the most advanced studies being performed on weight loss and health of the human body.

Dr. Luigi Fontana, professor at the Washington University in St. Louis, School of Medicine, was the first stop for Dr. Mosley. He learned that people with complete **low-calorie restriction**[2], known as CRONies[3] (Calorie Restriction with Optimal Nutrients), were extremely healthy. They gained a 50% increase in lifespan[4] and are "almost like another species"[5]. Dr. Mosley, excited to learn about longevity and aging, had a dilemma though; living on such a calorie-restricted diet was a drastic lifestyle change that he wasn't ready for.

Dr. Valter Longo, professor at the University of Southern California's School of Longevity, was next in Dr. Mosley's quest. Dr. Longo[6] had been testing the how fasting effects insulin-like growth factor-1 (IGF-1). [7] This growth factor, IGF-1, is a factor of aging as well as a prerequisite for cancer to develop.

When your body produces IGF-1, it makes your cells grow and reproduce, thus "ageing". When you fast, or restrict your calories for specific amounts of time, your liver goes into a "starvation" mode and does not create IGF-1 as much. At this point, your body no longer uses glucose for energy, going into a mode where it repairs unhealthy or damaged cells it needs to "survive".[8]

So, to summarize, when you give your body (and hormones) a break from calories and processed foods with the 5:2 method, then your body can begin to fix itself- or **live longer and healthier!** Does this sound too good to be true? Well, studies are showing that aging can be truly slowed in its progression when you go down to the mitochondrial[9] level of cells. The way you allow those cells to repair themselves is by allowing those IGF-1 levels to lower.[10]

Dr. Mosely spent 4 days fasting to test these studies. After fasting, his blood glucose levels and IGF-1 levels lowered tremendously. But, Dr. Mosley felt that fasting like this would be too hard. Even though prolonged fasting has great benefits, he did not feel as if the lifestyle would suit him or that he would consistently follow through. **He wanted a real change!**

Dr. Krista Varaday, a researcher in obesity at the University of Illinois-Chicago, was the next person Dr. Mosely spoke with. Varaday researches alternate day fasting, one day fasting (500 kcal), and then the next day eating whatever. Her studies were to determine the benefits of fasting on these alternate days to gather scientific data of weight loss, blood pressure, diabetes, and cholesterol.

Although, Varaday suggests every other day, Mosley found his method too constricting and chose to fast two days per week, Monday and Thursday, eating 600kcal on fasting days. He found this method to be much easier to do as a lifestyle than the constant calorie restriction or prolonged fasting. This 2 day fasting method is when he began to see the weight loss and his blood pressure, sugar levels, and cholesterol improve! Mosley knew that he could live this lifestyle- fasting 2 days per week. He tested this 5:2 day diet and was amazed at his results in just 5 weeks!

Dr. Michael Mosley's research, experience, and decision to live a healthy lifestyle, that worked for him, was the creation of the 5:2 diet! <u>My purpose is to help you get started, help you find meal plans that you enjoy, and show you the benefits of high-intensity exercise that will give you a longer and healthier life!</u> My true goal and passion is to motivate you and inspire you with my own success and experiences on the 5:2. Feel free to explore my <u>website</u> and download my 5:2-app to your smartphone (<u>Apple</u>, <u>Android</u>), to get the full benefit of the 5:2 lifestyle!

Now that you know about Dr. Mosley's quest, his research, and the celebratory lifestyle of 5:2, including my success and experience with it, you might be left with a few questions or concerns. Allow these following benefits to help guide you in making the best choice of your life! Just remember, don't use your non-fasting days as a reason to overeat. This is a new way of living healthy and living longer. Intermittent fasting with the use of calorie restriction, as well as high-intensity exercise, has many benefits. Let's take a look at the studies about these benefits so you can feel confident that 5:2 is for you! Please be advised that if you are pregnant, or an adolescent then you should not attempt 5:2 and if you are taking medications then you should speak to your physician.

Benefits

Now that you know about Dr. Mosley's quest, his research, and the celebratory lifestyle of 5:2, including my success and experience with it, you might be left with a few questions or concerns. Allow these following benefits help guide you in making the best choice of your life! Just remember, don't use your non-fasting days as a reason to overeat. This is a new way of living healthy and living longer. Intermittent fasting with the use of calorie restriction, as well as high-intensity exercise, has many benefits. Let's take a look at the studies about these benefits so you can feel confident that 5:2 is for you—the many benefits beyond weight loss!

Please be advised that if you are pregnant, or an adolescent then you should not attempt 5:2 and if you are taking medications then you should speak to your physician.

You can lower your risk (and possibly reverse):

- ✓ Stroke
- ✓ Blood Sugar
- ✓ Blood Fats (lipids)
- ✓ Cancer Formations
- ✓ Alzheimer's

- ✓ Heart Disease
- ✓ Insulin Levels
- ✓ Diabetes Type 2
- ✓ Kidney Disease
- ✓ Insulin Sensitivity

You can improve:

- ✓ Immunity
- ✓ Cardiovascular Health
- ✓ Resistance to Parkinson's
- ✓ Longevity (Aging)
- ✓ Brain Activity & Memory (protect against dementia)

This list of benefits may seem extraordinary- and they are! The science of intermittent fasting in not new, it's based on centuries of cultural observations, nutrition studies, and eating habits. The science and research is abundant and promising. Let me review some of the health benefits that can occur with 5:2!

Live Longer! Live Healthier! (with 5:2 diet)

5:2 is a method of intermittent fasting (or calorie restriction) where one would choose two days of the week to eat 500 or 600 calories depending on gender, 500 calories for females and 600 for males. As you know, the method of 5:2 was developed from the research of Dr. Mosley. Intermittent fating or calorie restriction is a way of changing your eating pattern.

People who have chosen these lifestyles have been studies for generations on the effects of such type of eating. A longer life span[11] has been noticed in those with calorie-restricted diets. One aspect of this longer life is the lower levels of oxidative stress, cellular repair that occurs which reduces aging, and insulin resistance. 5:2 can provide your body with greater immunity. The days of lower caloric needs allows the body to repair itself.

The effect of weight loss (especially abdominal fat that has shown to increase cardiovascular disease and Type 2 diabetes) allows for a lowering of triglycerides, which in turn improve cholesterol, plaque build-up in arteries[12], blood lipids, blood sugars, and thus preventing cardiovascular[13] diseases as well as kidney disease[14], diabetes[15], endocrine[16] stresses, cancers[17], and stroke[18]. As cell repair[19] increase the anti-aging effect does to. The cellular repair, restoration of insulin sensitivity, and reversal of adipose fat (belly weight), and protection of inflammation all contribute to these amazing benefits- even on your mood[20]!

Many studies have been taken in cultures where longevity is commonly found. For example, in ancient times when fasting was a part of religion as well as a part of restricted harvest and limited access to foods, the lower caloric dietary needs allowed for people to live longer. These facts warranted the research being done today based on the question; why do people live longer and healthier in third world countries and in ancient times than our diseased and early mortality rates of today? Click here[21] for a full study by Dr. Mosley on all these benefits and research.

With a lower calorie diet, one that is exemplary of 5:2 with its intermittent fasting, the ability for mental cognition enhances. Studies show that the brain[22] becomes more active, the ability to counter Alzheimer's[23] [24] increases, and the resistance to Parkinson's[25] increases too. The studies have been overwhelming with results in reference to how transformative calorie restriction is for the body in regards to reversal of disease and increase in resistance, beyond just simple weight loss, so much so that many more studies are in progress.

Mark Mattson[26], professor of neuroscience and Director of John Hopkins University in Baltimore says, " We're kicking off a pilot study of 20 women aged 55-70 who are at high risk of developing Alzheimer's." His studies have shown that a reduce in calories can keep the brain going which even protects against dementia; "The survival instinct compels us to keep going to eventually find food and brain activity in itself is believed to protect against dementia," explains Professor Mark Mattson. [27]

Future Studies in Progress

Furthermore, Professor Kerstin Bismar[28], Professor of Diabetes Research at the Department of Molecular Medicine and Surgery, who specializes in "diabetic complications, particularly the significance of the growth factor IGF-1 and its binding protein IGFBP-1, high blood sugar (hyperglycemia), shortage of oxygen (hypoxia), genetic factors and oxidative stress", has set in motion a study in which she will sample healthy people and type 2 diabetic patients that do the 5:2 diet. On my blog I will post the results as soon as I get access to them.

So, although testing on fasting and its benefits is still continuing, the research already conducted has compelling research and scientific studies thus far. Fasting diets will help you lose weight, especially if other diets have failed you because this is one that you will stick with! But wait! There is more to know...the 5:2 workout and why it is just as important to healthy living with the 5:2 diet. The 5:2 workout is based on high-intensity exercises.

Learn about the positive benefits of high-intensity exercise!

Follow my 5:2 workout to see the best benefits of high-intensity exercise!

The workouts are specifically targeted for the 5:2 diet. Check out my web app for more exercise!

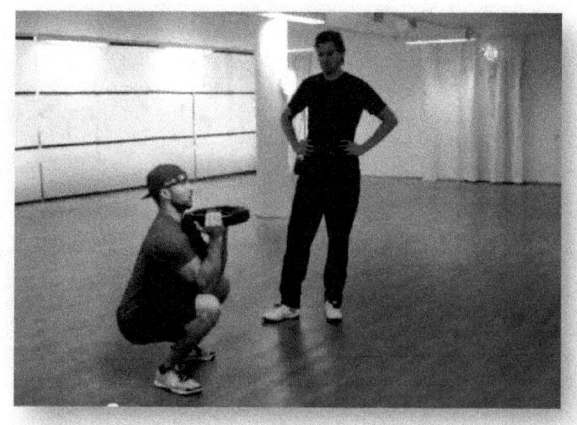

Live Longer! Live Healthier! (with 5:2 workout)

A sedentary life or over-consumption of calories can lead to weight gain. Weight gain, especially obesity, can lead to many types of risk factors[29] including heart disease, diabetes, high cholesterol, high blood pressure, cancers, and stroke. This is especially true in those aged 60+. For more information about 60+ plus, please scroll to the next section.

Once weight gain has set in, the ability to remove these risk factors can become a struggle. Diet and exercise is paramount to reversing health back to normal. Intermittent fasting is very powerful for weight loss along with exercising- specifically high-intensity exercise because it promotes greater shedding of body fat. Calorie restriction is necessary to lose weight but exercise is needed to lose substantial weight[30]. High-intensity exercise breaks burns more calories in less time and lasts longer throughout the day in regards to metabolic burn.

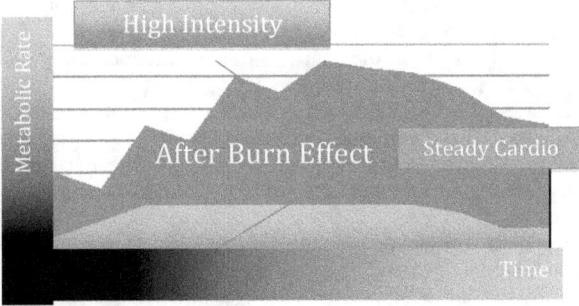

Your body benefits at a cellular level,[31] speeding up the process with bursts of exercise promotes a higher level of fat and glycogen breakdown. It has shown to progressively release fats in adipose tissues (belly fat) which has been shown to increase risks of cancers. You will improve insulin resistance[32] and sensitivity - possibly even reverse it! Insulin resistance has been linked to several types of cancer including breast, prostate and pancreatic cancers.

Blood pressure[33] improves with a combination of 5:2 and high-intensity exercise. You will gain glycemic control[34] in Type 2 diabetes, along with muscle strength. You will decrease oxidative radicals that damage cells, which in turn helps aging and disease. You will also reduce risk of stroke and improve cardiovascular health with high-intensity exercise[35].

 Studies show that the oxidation of fatty tissues (triglycerides) is actually different among gender[36]. Men have a harder time losing belly fat, a precursor to cancers and diseases, than women do. But, in fact, with fasting, men then get to experience the benefits for losing their belly fat combined with high-intensity exercise. The metabolic response[37] to exercise is increased with high-intensity training.

5:2 is a very safe and efficient method
allowing human beings to live a healthy, disease- free life.

Age 60+: Live Longer and Healthier, too!

If you are over the age of 60 and wondering if the benefits from 5:2 and high-intensity exercise will affect you, then be prepared, because yes they do!

High-intensity exercise is good for you, too! If you don't feel comfortable doing new exercises on land, then a good place to start is in the pool. Studies have shown that the buoyancy of water puts less stress on the joints and increases balance with the positive effects[38] of weight loss and health benefits. Also, high-intensity underwater running/jogging/aerobics has been determined to improve aerobic power[39] as well as improve[40] cardiovascular fitness, strength, and abdominal obesity in the overweight elderly.

Beyond weight loss, the health factors of 5:2 are incredible for those over 60—a phenomenon. The positive effects on the body are similar to those in younger people, almost reversing age with intramuscular, cardiovascular, and metabolic changes.[41] The increase of life span is a high motivator to begin your 5:2 diet. Longevity[42] has been well established with calorie-restricted lifestyles, as is evident by studies in Japan where people live on diet low in calories but rich in nutrients. Health benefits such as lower blood pressure[43] and memory improvement[44] in a diet with restricted calorie intake has proven to improve cognitive function in terms of memory as well as help maintain memory ability.

It is very important to note that if you are taking medication, then you should speak with your doctor. The health benefits of 5:2 and high-intensity exercise will only be a life-changing process for you—allowing you to live longer and live healthier!

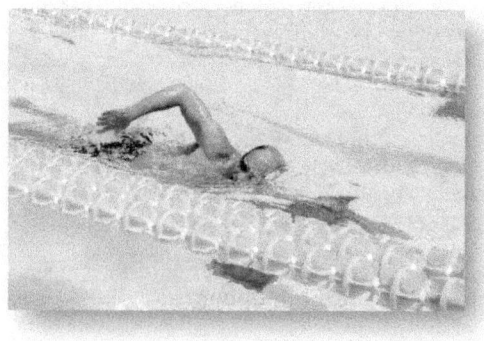

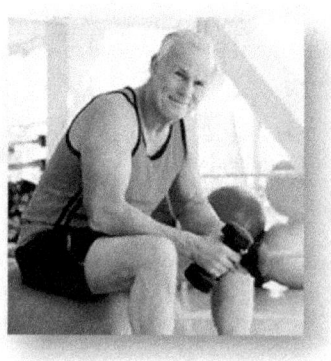

Side Effects

— Headache has been recorded during the first 2 weeks. I urge you to drink lots and lots of water. Drinking water usually subsides hunger as well as headaches—but this is a remedy even when not fasting! Also if you would get calf cramps at night, it's because you drank too little during the day. Also, be sure to salt/seasoning food well on fasting days.

Multiple studies show that drinking water can cure a headache for many reasons, so water should be your choice of drink -and drunk plenty- regardless of dieting! It is a must!

— Some have felt irritation the first few times of fast days. I myself felt it after the first day, but it passes.

— I've heard of some sleep problems in the media but none of my thousands of blog readers have mentioned it.

The first 2-3 weeks are the hardest and have the most side effects, but keep reminding yourself of all the benefits you will gain!

*In elderly people, calorie restriction has been indicative of osteoporosis, but...5:2 is not living a daily life of calorie restriction! For 5 days you have the freedom to eat plenty of healthy food. If you are still concerned, then you must know that many people above the age of 60 years live on completely calorie restricted diets- every day! These people prevent loss of bone mass and osteoporosis by walking 5k about 4-5 times per week as well as by getting plenty of sunshine, such as Bob Cavanaugh, 64, managing director of the Calorie Restriction Society International.[45] Studies conclude that nutrient rich diets prevent reduced bone minerals. Eating 5:2 actually helps you eat much healthier as on non-fasting days you begin to change to healthier eating too![46]

Who Shouldn't 5:2

Very Important!

Before starting with the 5:2 diet, it is good to consult your doctor if you take medications, are pregnant, or have long standing medical conditions such as eating disorders or obesity. Also, people under 18 years old should not do the 5:2 diet.

5:2 Basics

Start Easy

1. Start by selecting 2 days in the week that you will fast. ***Do not fast one day after the other.*** I chose to fast on Monday and Thursday like Dr. Mosley did.

2. Women eat 500 calories (kcal) on fast days. Men eat 600 calories (kcal).

3. On your fast days it is important that you ***eat healthy whole foods*** full of fiber, vitamins, and minerals. Eat clean! You should not use manufactured foods such as shakes, bars, or other processed foods. You are eating few calories, so make those calories count!

4. Hold down on the simple carbs on fasting days such as sugar, white bread, and white pasta. Refined carbohydrates are unhealthy. Check the ingredients for unbleached, unrefined wheat, grains, etc.

5. At least 20-25% of food should be protein on fast days. I recommend eating a high protein breakfast. See my exact recipe. My wife and I tested to find out the proper measurements for healthy proteins so you feel good and balanced during the day.

   * You can eat a normal diet the ordinary days but try not to overdo your protein intake. If you eat normal, then you will not over eat protein anyway, so you don't need to go and think about this all the time. Good protein is found in chicken, tuna, shrimp, plants, and eggs of course!

   Professor Valter Longo recommends 0.8 g of protein per kg of your body weight per day. For me, weighing 75 kg would be 0.8 x 75 = 60g.

   How to calculate:
   ✓ Divide your weight in lbs by 2.2 to find your weight in kg.
   ✓ Multiply your weight in kg by 0.8 to find your grams of protein per day.

$lbs \div 2.2 = kg$
$kg \times 0.8 = g \ of \ protein$

Example: 178 lbs ÷ 2.2 = 80.90
80.90 × 0.8 = 64.7 (65) grams of protein per day!

5:2 has become a lifestyle for me, or I will now say 6:1. You see, after 5 months I reached my target weight! So, I then started to fast only 1 day a week—Thursday. **6:1 is how to maintain!** I suggest you do 5:2 for 5 months, then switch to 6:1.

Once you reach 6:1, all the health benefits you have built up will remain AND keep your weight the same. Dr. Michael Mosley also does 6:1 now, too. After 5 months with 5:2, he started with 6:1. After a year with 6:1, he maintained his weight. All the tests he does regularly for his health shows that it's enough to just fast 1 day a week once you have done 5:2.

Tips to Succeed

➢ Wondering how and when to eat it on 5:2? There is one simple rule: The only thing you need to consider is to have your 500 calories during the day when you are awake. For example, you might think that you can start at 20.00 (8p.m.) on Sunday night, eat your calories the next morning, and then at 20.00 (8p.m.) Monday evening stop fasting and eat a big dinner! This type of schedule is not ideal. But, if that's the only way you can fit 5:2 in your lifestyle, then a lifestyle with 5:2 is still better than one without.

➢ Divide your 500 kcal or 600 kcal into 2 or 3 meals. *3 meals worked best for me!*

➢ Vitamin supplements are not needed; if you have been advised to take vitamins by a professional nutritionist then you should. But otherwise, I recommend not using it.

➢ You can drink coffee/tea without milk and sugar without counting the calories. But, be aware that it is a diuretic so you will still need to drink ordinary water. The body is used to getting water from food and on the fast days your body still needs that water.

➢ Drink up to 3 liters of water during the day. For lunch you can have a slice of lemon in the water for taste. If you don't drink enough water, you could get a headache and maybe some muscle cramps at night, for example, in the calf.

➢ A glass of water is the trick for hunger. Sometimes, people think they are hungry when they are really thirsty instead.

➢ **You can be flexible with 5:2!** Do you get invited for a night out on your scheduled fast day? Did you plan to fast on Monday but forgot about that football game? You can easily change your scheduled day. Don't get caught up too much in your scheduled day- just be careful not to fast two days in a row. For me, I now do 6:1; fasting just 1 day in the week means I can really be flexible. That's why I believe **this is for the long run!**

➢ Do you have holiday? You can do 6:1 instead of 5:2, or no fasting at all! Enjoy your holiday as much as you can. You can always go back to 5:2 or 6:1 afterwards. This is not a "fad diet". This is for the long run and you need to be comfortable in the lifestyle. Just be conscientious and don't over-eat.

➢ Fasting days are perfect opportunities to abstain from alcohol. I suggest not drinking alcohol on fast days.

➢ Adding a teaspoon of olive oil in salads (but deducting the calories) makes the fat-soluble vitamins in the salad more likely to be absorbed by the body. Add spices or herbs to liven the salad.

➢ Avoid using chewing gum during fasting days. It can trick your body a little bit.

How Quickly Will I See Results?

Your first two weeks can be quite annoying, as the body is not accustomed to the calorie restriction yet. My first 2 weeks were annoying! After the first day, I felt a bit annoyed but it was over quickly. I also drank too little water one day during those first weeks and got a cramp in the calf one night.

I tend to measure my waist at exactly the same place every time. I lie down on my back, relax, and take a tape measure around the navel. I usually do this every Monday morning. I weigh myself then, too.

- Expect that you lose about 0.4-0.5 kg (about 1lb) per week initially. Check out my progress here .

- Do not compare yourself with others. I lost 7 kg for the first 7 weeks because I completely committed to a better mindset and pulled down on the sweets. It is important not to think too much. Eat as usual during the five regular days. Just try to remember you are getting healthy, so *keep in mind 'everything in moderation'.* Be sensible. Over-eating will not lead to success.

- If you do not lose weight immediately, remember that you are not gaining weight and you are getting positive effects on your health!

- If you have a hard time one day, just think, "Tomorrow I'll eat that yummy sandwich for lunch!" The strength to know "tomorrow I can eat whatever I want," makes it much easier. In this way, I really think that 5:2 can become a way of life for most people.

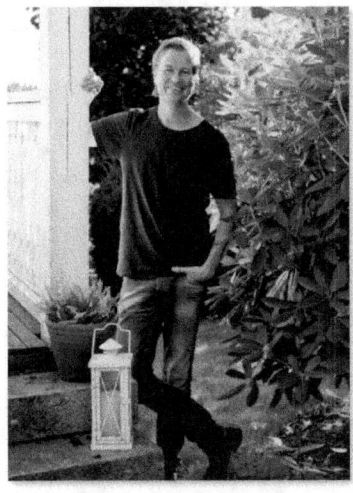

Hold out for the first 2-3 weeks; it feels really easy after that!

You deserve to be healthy!

5:2 is so simple, yet the benefits are extraordinary!

You'll love this diet because of the following reasons:

➤ No complicated rules to follow—flexible, understandable, and user friendly.
➤ No daily calorie counting. None of the tedious/frustrating methods of other diets.
➤ One cool thing: fasting activates countless repair genes and heals old cells.
➤ Yes, it is fasting, but not as you know it. You will not starve; only lower your calories for one day (two days in a week, but not consecutive).
➤ You'll still eat the food you love, most of the time.
➤ Once you reach your weight, you can run 6:1. Then the weight will not increase and you still get the health benefits.
➤ 5:2 - method is a viable strategy for a healthy and long life.

Other ways to get in some exercise- you won't believe!

✓ Stand while you use the telephone or maybe a few times when you watch television. Maybe do some exercise or lift hand-weights while watching television. Make yourself do 5 minutes of push-ups or sit-ups before turning on the TV.
✓ While watching TV, lift lightweights to incorporate more strength-building exercises into your day.
✓ Clean your house! Wash windows, sweep, and do laundry! Even move furniture. All moving is good for you. When doing laundry, do some leg squats with the laundry basket full.
✓ Use a bathroom on another level, upstairs or downstairs so you can use the stairs! You can do this anywhere!
✓ Stretch in the morning and at night. **Wake up and do 5 minutes of crunches/push up.**
✓ Park your car far away from your destination so you can walk.
✓ Avoid the drive-thru; instead walk inside.
✓ Instead of playing cards or going to dinner with friends, bike ride, of take a walk through the woods.
✓ Garden.
✓ Play in park. Ride a bicycle. Wrestle with the children! Have fun and be active.
✓ Walk errands; walk quickly!
✓ Get a pedometer! Track how many step you take. When you see how many you take in a day, then you may decide to take more!
✓ When waiting in line, flex your abs 10 sec/repeat 10 times. No one can see!
✓ Lift cans, lift laundry detergent; use your groceries for weight lifting while putting them away! Carry bags from the store to your car or carry them several times to your home- do some sprints! It'll only take a few minutes more.
✓ Take the stairs instead of the elevator.
✓ Ride the bus then get off early and walk the rest of the way park farther away.
✓ Don't email or phone, walk or go visit your friends.
✓ Wash car by hand.
✓ Walk on weekends. Take a long walk.
✓ Walk your dog twice!

Menus

Use my 5:2-app (<u>Apple</u>, <u>Android</u>) and use these recipes in the kitchen or when you are at the store! Recipes have conversions. If you would like more conversions please click for <u>weight</u> and <u>volume</u>. Remember the <u>5:2 Basics</u>!

Tips:

* A large cup of organic green tea in the evening (no milk or sugar) helps hunger and counts as 0kcal. Green tea is very good for you! Also, a few cups of black coffee during the day counts as 0 kcal (no sugar or milk).
* Drink plenty of water during the day about 3 liters .
* Cold water with lime is really good.
* Please take a little sea salt in plain water during the day.

(Warning- fizzy drinks or plain water with lemon/lime is not so good for your teeth! Given that many people today have trouble with sensitive teeth and enamel weakening, I suggest just drinking these drinks with your food and remember to always drink water!)

Meal Plan #1

Breakfast:
* ICA's quark   10% fat: 50 g (1.7 oz.)= 0.50x140 = 84 kcal *Quark is like cottage cheese.
* Mild yoghurt   0.5% fat: 1.6 dl (1/4 cup) = 1.6 x40 = 64 kcal
* Cinnamon: 0 kcal

Mix in a little vanilla powder, for a yummy treat.

Total: 148 kcal

Lunch:
Hamburgers & Dressing

* Ground Beef   10% fat: 500 grams (1.1 lb)= 5x149 = 745 kcal
* 1 clove of garlic   about 5 grams (.17 oz.)=0.05 x158 = ~ 8kcal
* 1 egg, normal sized   77 kcal
* Butter   about 5 grams (1 tsp or .17oz) = 0.05 X720 = 36 kcal
* Salt
* White Pepper
* Black Pepper

Chop the garlic and mix together with the egg and ground beef. Mince well. Add salt and pepper. Form 5 patties to make burgers at about 100 grams (3.5 oz.) each. Fry them in butter. Sprinkle black pepper and salt when it turns brown.

Total: 173 kcal (for hamburgers)

*Make your own dressing for the hamburger with sour cream and chili sauce or flavored ketchup seasoned with a little white pepper. Mix 4 tablespoons sour cream (about 100 grams or 3.5 ounces, 1x140 = 140 kcal), with 1 tablespoon chili sauce or flavored ketchup (about 20 grams or 0.7 ounces, 0.2 x 100 = 20 kcal). Total calories in the dressing become 160 kcal (5 servings).

- Dressing   1 Tablespoon = 160/5 = 32 kcal
- Romaine Lettuce   20 grams (0.7 oz.) = 0.2x15 = 3 kcal
- Red onion   10 grams (0.35 oz.)= 0.1x35 = 3.5 kcal
- 1 Tomato   100 grams (3.5 oz.)= 1x26 = 26kcal
- Cucumber   20 grams (0.7 oz.) = 0.2x11 = 2.2 kcal

Use romaine lettuce as "hamburger bread," with one leaf for the bottom and one for the top. It is crunchy, easy to eat, and delicious! Add the hamburger between your "lettuce bread" and add the red onion, salad dressing, tomato and cucumber.

Total: 173 kcal (for dressing)

Total for lunch: 240 kcal

Dinner:
Men
- 2 eggs   77 kcal x 2 = 144 kcal
- Finn Crisp Original (3 plates)   20 kcal x 3 = 60 kcal *Finn Crips are whole-grain rye crackers

Women
- 1 egg   77 kcal
- 2 Finn Crisp original (2 plates)   20 kcal x 2 = 40 kcal

Total: 204 kcal (men)
*   127 kcal (women)*

Total for Meal Plan #1 = 505 kcal (women) 592 kcal (men)

Meal Plan #2

Breakfast:
- 1 egg (may add salt)   77 kcal
- Frozen Blueberry   *Women 25 g (0.88 oz.) = 0.25 x 55 = 14 kcal
      *Men   50 g (1.6 oz.) = 0.50 x 55 = 28 kcal
- Frozen Raspberries   *Women 25 g (0.88 oz.) = 0.25 x 47 = 12 kcal
      *Men   50 g (1.6 oz.) = 0.50 x 47 = 23 kcal
- Tea/Coffee   0 kcal
  (no milk or sugar)

Total: 103 kcal (women)
*   128 kcal (men)*

Lunch:
- Mozzarella   60 g (2.11oz.) = 0.60 × 251 = 150.6 kcal
- Cherry Tomatoes   100 g (3.5 oz.) = 1.0 × 26 = 26 kcal
- Olive Oil   1 teaspoon = 0.027 × 900 = 25 kcal
- Onion   20 g (0.7 oz.) = 0.20 × 35 = 7 kcal
- Cashews   *Women 7 g (0.25 oz.)= 0.07 x 610 = 42.7 kcal
      *Men 19 g (0.7 oz.)= .19 x 610 = 116 kcal
- Fresh Basil   5g (0.17 oz.) = 0.05 × 25 = about 1.3 kcal
- Apple Cider Vinegar   5g (0.17 oz.) = 0.05 × 15 = about 1 kcal

Plate nicely and season with salt (sea salt is great!). Fresh basil can be substituted with iceberg lettuce.

Total: 254 kcal (women)
*   327 kcal (men)*

Dinner:
- Salmon   40 g (1.4 oz.) = 0.40 × 230 = 92 kcal
- Broccoli   60 g (2.1 oz.) = 0.60 × 25 = 15 kcal
- Carrot   60 g (2.1 oz.) = 0.60 × 31 = about 19 kcal
- Tomato   40 g (1.4 oz.) = 0.40 × 26 = approx 10.4 kcal
- Bell Pepper (red)   20 g (0.7 oz.) = 0.20x36 = about 7.2 kcal

Preheat the oven to 225 degrees and season the salmon with lemon pepper.
Next, add in broccoli , sliced carrots, sliced tomato, and shredded pepper .
Let everything cook in the oven for 15 minutes. Season with a little sea salt on everything.
Weigh, after all, been in the oven. Add in a little more than you think the first time so you can find the right process.

Total: 143 kcal

Total for the Meal Plan #2 = 500 kcal (women) 598 kcal (men)

Meal Plan #3

___

Breakfast:
- 1 egg (may salt egg)   77 kcal
- 1 slice FINN CRISP   20 kcal
- Frozen Great Blueberry ICA   25 g (0.88 oz.) = 0.50 x 55 = about 28 kcal
- Tea/Coffee   0 kcal
  (no milk and sugar)

Total: 97 kcal (women)
        125 kcal (men)

Lunch:
- Mozzarella   60 g (2.1 oz.) = 0.60 × 251 = 150.6 kcal
- Cherry Tomatoes   100g (3.5 oz.) = 1.0 × 26 = 26 kcal
- Olive Oil   1 teaspoon = 0.027 × 900 = 25 kcal
- Onion   20 g (0.7 oz.) = 0.20 × 35 = 7 kcal *choose yellow, white, or red onion
- Cashews   *Women 7 grams (0.25 oz.) = 0.07 x 610 = about 42.7 kcal
                          *Men 19 g = 116 kcal)
- Fresh Basil   5g (0.18 oz.) = 0.05 × 25 = about 1.3 kcal * iceburg lettuce substitution
- Apple Cider Vinegar   5 g (0.18 oz.) = 0.05 × 15 = about 1 kcal

Add ingredients up nicely and season with herbal salt or sea salt .

Total: 254 kcal (women)
        327 kcal (men)

Dinner:
- 2 cups Mild light yogurt   2 cups = 40 Kcal
- Apple Slices   110 g (3.9 oz.) = 1.1 × 60 = 66 kcal

Slice apple into pieces and season with cinnamon as it is good and healthy.

Total: 146 kcal

Total for the Meal Plan #3 = 497 kcal (women) 598 kcal (men)

Meal Plan #4

Breakfast:
- 1 egg (may salt egg)   77 kcal
- Frozen Blueberries   *Women 70 g (2.5 oz.) = 0.70x55 = 38.5 kcal
  -      *Men 110 g (3.9 oz.) = 60.5 kcal
- Tea/Coffee   0 kcal
  (no milk or sugar)

Total: 115.5 kcal (women)
*   138 kcal (men)*

Lunch:
- Mixed salad ICA   30g (1 oz.) = 0.30 × 18 = 5.4 kcal
- Goji Berries   5 g (0.18 oz.) = 0.05 × 313 = 15.5 Kcal
- Onion   20g (0.7 oz.) = 0.20 × 35 = 7 kcal
- Watermelon   100g (3.5 oz.) = 1.0 × 40 = 40 kcal
- Feta Cheese (Apertina Arla, classic)   50 g (1.8 oz.) = 0.5 × 215 = 108 kcal
- Olive Oil   1 teaspoon = 0.027 × 900 = 25 kcal

Create a mixed salas with ingredients. Add feta chesse and oil to top, add oregeno for spice.

Total: 201 kcal

Dinner:
- Chicken   80 g (2.8 oz.) = 0.8 × 115 = about 92 kcal
- Salted Cashews   *Women 10 g (0.35 oz.) = 0.10 × 610 = approx. 61 kcal
  -      *Men 20 g (0.7 oz.) = 0.20 × 610 = approx. 122 kcal
- Carrots   50 g (1.8 oz.) = 0.50 × 31 = approx. 15.5 kcal
- Cherry Tomatoes   30 g (1.06 oz.) = 0.30 × 26 = about 8 kcal
  -      50 g (1.8 oz.) = 0.30 x 26 = about 13 kcal
- Orange Peppers   *Women 20g (0.7 oz.) = 0.20 × 0.3 = 6 kcal
  -      *Men 50 g (1.8 oz.) = 0.50 x 0.3 = 15 kcal

Season the chicken with oregano and herbal salt.

Total: 183 kcal (women)
*   258 kcal (men)*

Total for the Meal Plan #4 = 499.5 kcal (women) 597 kcal (men)

Meal Plan #5

Breakfast:
- 1 egg (may salt egg)   77 kcal
- Frozen Blueberries   *Women 70 g (2.5 oz.) = 0.70x55 = 38.5 kcal
                        *Men 110 g (3.9 oz.) = 60.5 kcal
- Tea/Coffee   0 kcal
     (no milk and sugar)

Total: 115.5 kcal (women)
*   132 kcal (men)*

Lunch:
- Cherry Tomatoes/Regular Tomatoes   200 g (7.05 oz.) = 2 × 0:26 = 52 kcal
- Goji berries   20 g (0.7 oz.) = 0.2 × 313 = 63 kcal
- Baby Spinach   65 g (2.3 oz.) = 0.65 × 15 = 10 kcal
- Pistachio Nuts   *Women 15 g (0.53oz.) = 0.15 × 610 = 91 kcal
                        *Men 20 g (0.7 oz.) = 0.20 x 610 = 122 kcal)

Total: 216 kcal (women)
*   247 kcal (men)*

Dinner:
- Iceberg lettuce   100 g (3.5 oz.) = 1.0 × 14 = approx. 14 kcal
- Chicken   50 g (1.8 oz.) = 0.5 × 115 = approx. 58 kcal
- Black Fiber Pasta   *Women 70 g (2.5 oz.) = 0.7 × 135 = about 95 kcal
                   *Men 110 g (3.9 oz.) = 0.7 x 3.9 = 148 kcal

(Note: Weigh pasta after you've cooked it for the 135 kcal. The pasta swells during cooking and the kcals would not be correct. 100 g of uncooked pasta is 365 kcal.

Total: 167 kcal (women)
*   220 kcal (men)*

Total for the Meal Plan #5 = 498.5 kcal (women) 599 kcal (men)

Workouts

To help you reach your goals and **become healthier and stronger**, I have created an exercise program with my personal trainer, Michael Hansson Sjöö. *We call it the 5:2 Workout.* This can be found on the web (http://myapp.is/52workout) so you can have it on any device as well as in this eBook.

- This is a system that consists of three exercise sessions per week, called "passes".
- The passes are short and highly intensive. They include heart rate-based strength training.

The workout names are in quotes- for example, the workout named "10-1". This is good to remember as you begin for future reference. A great thing to do is to print these next pages, cut out each Pass, and use them for reference.

My <u>website</u> is designed to help you with your dieting and exercise needs on 5:2. <u>Allow me to inspire you!</u>

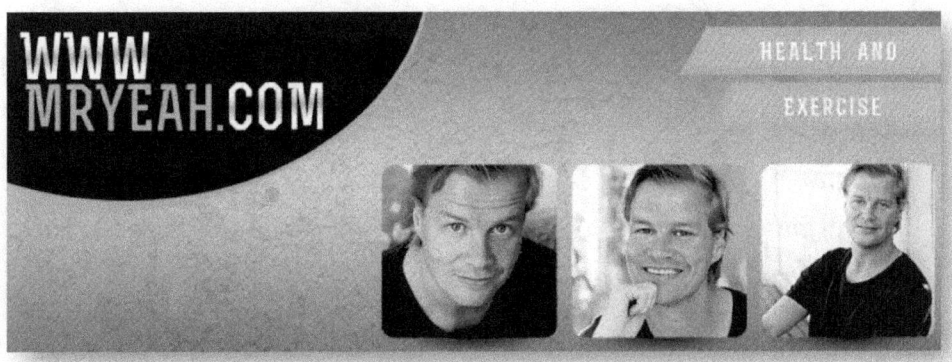

Week 1

Pass 1. "10-1" (You need to have the digital document so you can click and watch each exercise below)

- ✓ In n Out Push up
- ✓ Frog jumps
- ✓ Burpees

This pass consists of 3 exercises that happen in a rotation of 10 laps. During the first laps, do 10 repetitions of each exercise, the second lap 9 of each, the third lap becomes 8 of each, and so on, until you make the last lap which will then consist of only one repetition of each exercise--hence the name, "10-1", because you go from 10 repetitions to 1.

Write down the time it takes for you do the whole pass.

Pass 2. "3x5"

- ✓ 5 minutes Pushups
- ✓ Resting 2 minutes
- ✓ 5 minutes Air squats
- ✓ Resting 2 minutes
- ✓ 5 minutes Swing weight plate

This pass consists of 3 '5 minute intervals' made of 3 different exercises, hence "3x5". You then do as many reps of the given exercises as possible. Rest 2 minutes between exercises.

Write down the number of repetitions you got on each exercise.

Pass 3. "550"

- ✓ 100 Squats Fitness ball
- ✓ 90 Jumping jacks
- ✓ 80 GTO Ground to overhead (weight plate)
- ✓ 70 Saxjumps
- ✓ 60 Dips
- ✓ 50 In n Outs
- ✓ 40 Step forward
- ✓ 30 Torso twist
- ✓ 20 Parachutes
- ✓ 10 Burpees

This pass consists of 550 repetitions, hence the name "550". Work your way through with a good pace and as little rest as possible.

Write down the time it takes for you to do the whole pass.

Week 2

Pass 1. "20-15-10"

- ✓ 20 Handplants
- ✓ 15 Shaft presses weight plate
- ✓ 10 Frog jumps

This pass consists of 3 exercises conducted in the given number, over and over again for 15 minutes. Try to do as many laps as possible in the 15 minutes—15 minutes max!

Write down the number of laps you have done during your 15 minutes.

Pass 2. "20-10"

- ✓ 20 Mountain climbers
- ✓ 10 Dips

This pass consists of only 2 exercises but performed for 10 laps.

Write down the time it takes you to do it all.

Pass 3. "10-20-30"

- ✓ 10 Thrusters weight plate
- ✓ 20 Sax jumps
- ✓ 30 Meatballs

This pass runs for 5 laps and consists of 3 exercises that are done in the given number of repetitions during each lap.

Write down the time it takes for you to do it all.

Week 3

Pass 1. "10-1, 1-10"

- ✓ <u>Plate squat</u>
- ✓ <u>Swing weight plate</u>
- ✓ <u>Parachutes</u>

This session consists of three exercises and performed by 20 laps.
You start at 10 and go down to 1 repetition. Than you go from 1 up to 10 again.

Write down the time it takes for you to do this pass.

Pass 2. "20x5"

- ✓ 5 <u>In n Outs</u>
- ✓ 5 <u>Jumpsquats</u>
- ✓ 5 <u>Pushups</u>

This pass includes a 20-minute workout and 3 exercises. You do 5 repetitions of each exercise during the entire session.

Write down the maximum number of laps you did in 20 minutes.

Pass 3. "3x5"

- ✓ 5 minutes <u>Bulgarian split squat</u> right leg
- ✓ Resting 2 minutes
- ✓ 5 minutes <u>Bulgarian split squat</u> left leg
- ✓ Resting 2 minutes
- ✓ 5 minutes <u>Hindu pushup</u>

This workout consists of two exercises. 1 exercise runs in two innings (on each leg). In five minutes, you should gather as many reps as you can.

Note the number of reps you did in 5 minutes.

Week 4

Pass 1. "300"

- ✓ 100 Dips
- ✓ 100 Saxjumps
- ✓ 100 Plank with leg lift

This pass consisting of 300 reps split over 3 exercises. When you reach 100 repetitions of the first exercise, go to the second exercise, and then finish with 100 rep on the third.

Write down the time it takes for you to implement it all.

Pass 2. "3x2"

- ✓ 3 minutes Step forward
- ✓ Resting 2 minutes
- ✓ 3 minutes Pushups
- ✓ Resting 2 minutes
- ✓ 3 minutes Swing weight plate
- ✓ Resting 2 minutes

This pass consists of 3 exercises running over 3 minutes and 2 laps. Rest two minutes between the exercises.

Note the number of repetitions you can make.

Pass 3. "Go 50!"

- ✓ 50 Plate squat
- ✓ 50 Roll Outs Fitness ball
- ✓ 50 Thrusters weight plate
- ✓ 50 Meatballs
- ✓ 50 Jumping Jacks
- ✓ 50 Pushups

This class consists of all 6 exercises with 50 repetitions on each.

Write down the time it takes you to do it all.

[1] Mosley, Michael Dr. "Eat, Fast, and Live Longer." BBC. Horizon Films. 2012. http://vimeo.com/54089463 http://www.bbc.co.uk/programmes/p00wzndg

[2] Fontana, Luigi, Manlio Vinciguerra, and Valter D. Longo. "Growth factors, nutrient signaling, and cardiovascular aging." *Circulation research* 110.8 (2012): 1139-1150. http://circres.ahajournals.org/content/110/8/1139.short

[3] Cava, Edda, and Luigi Fontana. "Will calorie restriction work in humans?." *Aging (Albany NY)* 5.7 (2013): 507. http://www.ncbi.nlm.nih.gov/pmc/articles/PMC3765579/

[4] "Dr. Luigi Fontana Explores Caloric Restriction." *American Federation for Aging Research : News*. Health Research Alliance, 11 Feb. 2010. http://www.afar.org/news/view/dr-luigi-fontana-explores-caloric-restriction

[5] Mosley, Michael Dr. "Eat, Fast, and Live Longer." BBC. Horizon Films. 2012. http://vimeo.com/54089463 http://www.bbc.co.uk/programmes/p00wzndg

[6] V. D. Longo - Evidence for Programmed Aging. http://www.programmed-aging.org/theory-3/longo.html

[7] Parrella, Edoardo, and Valter D. Longo. "Insulin/IGF-I and related signaling pathways regulate aging in nondividing cells: from yeast to the mammalian brain." *The Scientific World Journal* 10 (2010): 161-177. http://www.hindawi.com/journals/tswj/2010/727632/abs/ http://www.ncbi.nlm.nih.gov/pubmed/20098959

[8] Mosley, Michael Dr. "Eat, Fast, and Live Longer." BBC. Horizon Films. 2012. http://vimeo.com/54089463 http://www.bbc.co.uk/programmes/p00wzndg

[9] Guarente, Leonard. "Mitochondria—a nexus for aging, calorie restriction, and sirtuins?." *Cell* 132.2 (2008): 171-176. http://www.sciencedirect.com/science/article/pii/S0092867408000627

[10] V. D. Longo - Evidence for Programmed Aging. http://www.programmed-aging.org/theory-3/longo.html

[11] Fontana, Luigi, Linda Partridge, and Valter D. Longo. "Dietary Restriction, Growth Factors and Aging: from yeast to humans." *Science (New York, NY)* 328.5976 (2010): 321. http://www.ncbi.nlm.nih.gov/pmc/articles/PMC3607354/

[12] Fontana, Luigi, et al. "Long-term calorie restriction is highly effective in reducing the risk for atherosclerosis in humans." *Proceedings of the National Academy of Sciences of the United States of America* 101.17 (2004): 6659-6663. http://www.pnas.org/content/101/17/6659.short

[13] Eshghinia and Mohammadzadeh Journal of Diabetes & Metabolic Disorders 2013, 12:4
http://www.jdmdonline.com/content/12/1/4

[14] Börgeson, Emma, and Kumar Sharma. "Obesity, immunomodulation and chronic kidney disease." *Current opinion in pharmacology* (2013).
http://www.sciencedirect.com/science/article/pii/S1471489213000714

[15] Azevedo, Fernanda Reis de, Dimas Ikeoka, and Bruno Caramelli. "Effects of intermittent fasting on metabolism in men." *Revista da Associação Médica Brasileira* 59.2 (2013): 167-173. http://www.scielo.br/scielo.php?pid=S0104-42302013000200017&script=sci_arttext&tlng=pt

[16] Azevedo, Fernanda Reis de, Dimas Ikeoka, and Bruno Caramelli. "Effects of intermittent fasting on metabolism in men." *Revista da Associação Médica Brasileira* 59.2 (2013): 167-173. http://www.scielo.br/scielo.php?pid=S0104-42302013000200017&script=sci_arttext&tlng=pt

[17] Anson, R. Michael, et al. "Intermittent fasting dissociates beneficial effects of dietary restriction on glucose metabolism and neuronal resistance to injury from calorie intake." *Proceedings of the National Academy of Sciences* 100.10 (2003): 6216-6220.
http://www.ncbi.nlm.nih.gov/pmc/articles/PMC156352/#__ffn_sectitle

[18] Liu, Ai-Jun, et al. "Involvement of arterial baroreflex in the protective effect of dietary restriction against stroke." *Journal of Cerebral Blood Flow & Metabolism* (2013).
http://www.nature.com/jcbfm/journal/v33/n6/full/jcbfm201328a.html

[19] Kitada, Munehiro, et al. "Calorie restriction in overweight males ameliorates obesity-related metabolic alterations and cellular adaptations through anti-aging effects, possibly including AMPK and SIRT1 activation." *Biochimica et Biophysica Acta (BBA)-General Subjects* 1830.10 (2013): 4820-4827.
http://www.sciencedirect.com/science/article/pii/S0304416513002742

[20] Fond, Guillaume, et al. "Fasting in mood disorders: neurobiology and effectiveness. A review of the literature." *Psychiatry research* (2013).
http://www.sciencedirect.com/science/article/pii/S0165178112008153

[21] Brown, James E., Michael Mosley, and Sarah Aldred. "Intermittent fasting: a dietary intervention for prevention of diabetes and cardiovascular disease?." *The British Journal of Diabetes & Vascular Disease* 13.2 (2013): 68-72. http://bjdvd.com/content/13/2/68.full

[22] Martin, Bronwen, Mark P. Mattson, and Stuart Maudsley. "Caloric restriction and intermittent fasting: two potential diets for successful brain aging." *Ageing research reviews* 5.3 (2006): 332-353.
http://www.sciencedirect.com/science/article/pii/S1568163706000523

[23] Puglielli, Luigi. "Aging of the brain, neurotrophin signaling, and Alzheimer's disease: is IGF1-R the common culprit?." *Neurobiology of aging* 29.6 (2008): 795-811.

http://www.sciencedirect.com/science/article/pii/S0197458007000127

[24] Parrella, Edoardo, et al. "Protein restriction cycles reduce IGF-1 and phosphorylated Tau, and improve behavioral performance in an Alzheimer's disease mouse model." *Aging cell* (2013). http://onlinelibrary.wiley.com/doi/10.1111/acel.12049

[25] Anson, R. Michael, et al. "Intermittent fasting dissociates beneficial effects of dietary restriction on glucose metabolism and neuronal resistance to injury from calorie intake." *Proceedings of the National Academy of Sciences* 100.10 (2003): 6216-6220. http://www.ncbi.nlm.nih.gov/pmc/articles/PMC156352/#_ffn_sectitle

[26] Mark P. Mattson, PhD. Chief of Laboratory of Neurosciences, National Institute on Aging Professor, Department of Neuroscience, Johns Hopkins University School of Medicine http://neuroscience.jhu.edu/MarkMattsonrecentpapers.php

[27] Martin, Bronwen, Mark P. Mattson, and Stuart Maudsley. "Caloric restriction and intermittent fasting: two potential diets for successful brain aging." *Ageing research reviews* 5.3 (2006): 332-353. http://www.sciencedirect.com/science/article/pii/S1568163706000523

[28] Kerstin Brismar. Professor of Diabetes Research at the Department of Molecular Medicine and Surgery. Karolinska Institutet. http://ki.se/ki/jsp/polopoly.jsp?d=1943&l=en

[29] Kim, Kwang-Il, and Cheol-Ho Kim. "Calorie Restriction in the Elderly People." *Journal of Korean medical science* 28.6 (2013): 797-798. http://synapse.koreamed.org/DOIx.php?id=10.3346/jkms.2013.28.6.797

[30] Groven, Karen Synne, and Gunn Engelsrud. "Dilemmas in the process of weight reduction: Exploring how women experience training as a means of losing weight." *International journal of qualitative studies on health and well-being* 5.2 (2010).http://www.ncbi.nlm.nih.gov/pmc/articles/PMC2875968/

[31] Shiraev, Tim, and Gabriella Barclay. "Evidence based exercise." (2012).
[32] Babraj, John A., et al. "Extremely short duration high intensity interval training substantially improves insulin action in young healthy males." *BMC Endocrine Disorders* 9.1 (2009): 3. http://www.biomedcentral.com/1472-6823/9/3/

[33] Paoli, Antonio, et al. "Effects of high-intensity circuit training, low-intensity circuit training and endurance training on blood pressure and lipoproteins in middle-aged overweight men." *Lipids in health and disease* 12.1 (2013): 131. http://www.lipidworld.com/content/12/1/131

[34] Dunstan, David W., et al. "High-intensity resistance training improves glycemic control in older patients with type 2 diabetes." *Diabetes care* 25.10 (2002): 1729-1736. http://care.diabetesjournals.org/content/25/10/1729.long

[35] Shiraev, Tim, and Gabriella Barclay. "Evidence based exercise." (2012).

http://www.ncbi.nlm.nih.gov/pubmed/23210120

[36]Horowitz, Jeffrey F., et al. "Effect of endurance training on lipid metabolism in women: a potential role for PPARα in the metabolic response to training." *American Journal of Physiology-Endocrinology And Metabolism* 279.2 (2000): E348-E355. http://ajpendo.physiology.org/content/279/2/E348

[37] Babraj, John A., et al. "Extremely short duration high intensity interval training substantially improves insulin action in young healthy males." *BMC Endocrine Disorders* 9.1 (2009): 3. http://www.ncbi.nlm.nih.gov/pubmed/18362686

[38] Bergamin, Marco, et al. "Water-versus land-based exercise in elderly subjects: effects on physical performance and body composition." *Clinical interventions in aging* 8 (2013): 1109. http://www.ncbi.nlm.nih.gov/pmc/articles/PMC3762608/

[39] Broman, Gi, et al. "High intensity deep water training can improve aerobic power in elderly women." European journal of applied physiology 98.2 (2006): 117-123. http://link.springer.com/article/10.1007/s00421-006-0237-2#page-1

[40] Legge, M., L. Jones, and K. Meredith-Jones. "Circuit based deep water running improves cardiovascular fitness, strength and abdominal obesity in older, overweight women aquatic exercise intervention in older adults." http://bmsi.ru/doc/1bf3d0e8-1cb0-4bbf-8648-0cdbbebbbbbc

[41] Hagerman, Fredrick C., et al. "Effects of high-intensity resistance training on untrained older men. I. Strength, cardiovascular, and metabolic responses." *The Journals of Gerontology Series A: Biological Sciences and Medical Sciences* 55.7 (2000): B336-B346 http://biomedgerontology.oxfordjournals.org/content/55/7/B336.short

[42] Kim, Kwang-Il, and Cheol-Ho Kim. "Calorie Restriction in the Elderly People." *Journal of Korean medical science* 28.6 (2013): 797-798. http://synapse.koreamed.org/DOIx.php?id=10.3346/jkms.2013.28.6.797

[43] Santana, Hugo, et al. "The higher exercise intensity and the presence of allele I of ACE gene elicit a higher post-exercise blood pressure reduction and nitric oxide release in elderly women: an experimental study." *BMC cardiovascular disorders* 11.1 (2011): 71. http://www.ncbi.nlm.nih.gov/pmc/articles/PMC3261092/

[44] Witte, A. V., et al. "Caloric restriction improves memory in elderly humans." *Proceedings of the National Academy of Sciences* 106.4 (2009): 1255-1260. http://www.pnas.org/content/106/4/1255.short

[45] Morelle, Rebecca. BBC News. "Extreme dieting: Eat less, live longer?" http://news.bbc.co.uk/2/hi/science/nature/6617113.stm

[46] Villareal, Dennis T., et al. "Reduced bone mineral density is not associated with significantly reduced bone quality in men and women practicing long-term calorie

restriction with adequate nutrition." *Aging cell* 10.1 (2011): 96-102.http://www.ncbi.nlm.nih.gov/pmc/articles/PMC3607368/#_ffn_sectitle

Photo. Elderly swimming. Nathan Pfau. Flckr Creative Commons. Fort Rucker. Photo. Some Rights Reserved.

Photo. Eldery Exercise. By National Institutes of Health [Public domain], via Wikimedia Commons. http://commons.wikimedia.org/wiki/File%3AElderly_exercise.jpg